Praise for I Am A M...

MW01041988

"Micheal D. Mann clearly and ~~frankly describes his disability~~ diagnoses, the challenges they pose and the ways he has dealt with them. I Am a Man Who Cries overflows with incredible creativity. Mann excels as an essayist, a poet, a rapper, a storyteller and a wry humourist.

From his poem The Sun of Love:
  Love is like a donut.
  It's there
  Then it's gone.

This is a groundbreaking book, well written, and a totally enjoyable read. Micheal has not "transcended" FASD or any of his other "disabilities." Instead he is at one with himself. His work is of universal appeal and significance. " - David Roche

David Roche is an inspirational humorist, motivational speaker and performer. His first book is The Church of 80% Sincerity. He is now touring internationally with a show called "Catholic Erotica".

"This is a wonderful first book for Micheal, a powerful testament to his growth as both a writer and individual. It's great to have his old and new writing together in one collection, offering his humour, anger, and soulful insights about a life rich, raw, and loving. I applaud Micheal's courage and willingness to share with such sensitivity his triumph over addiction and other challenges. I still remember his fierce talent and charge when he read early rap poems. It has been an honour to be part of Micheal's writing life and to witness this success. " - Heather Conn

Heather Conn is an author, editor, and writing coach who has written for more than 50 publications. She co-authored Vancouver's Glory Years. Her latest book is the popular children's story Gracie's Got a Secret. She also gives workshops in Soul Collage.

I Am a Man Who Cries

Micheal D. Mann

To Audrey,

continue to inspire!! ☺

From Micheal

I Am A Man

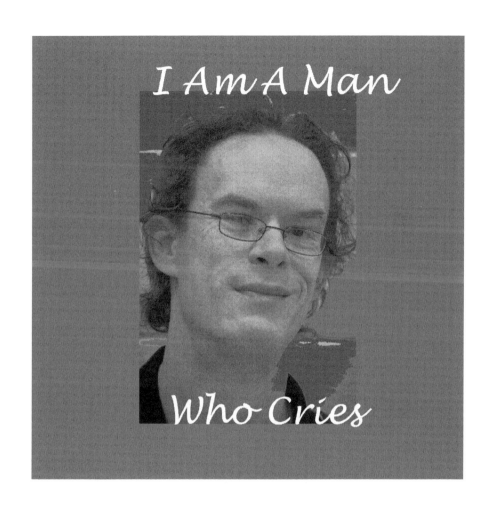

Who Cries

Micheal D. Mann

Calendula Farms

Library and Archives Canada Cataloguing in
Publication

Mann, Micheal D., 1982-
    I am a man who cries / Micheal D. Mann.

ISBN 978-0-9682477-2-3

    1. Mann, Micheal D., 1982-. 2. Fetal alcohol
syndrome--Patients--Canada--Biography. I. Title.

RG629.F45M29 2012   618.3'268610092   C2012-
904083-5

Book design by Jane Covernton
Cover, page 9, page 154 photos by Dominic Brooks.
Cover, page 138, page 154 photos by Laurie Kyle.
Back cover photo, photo page 42 by Sarju Sooch.
All other photos courtesy Helen Halet.
Detail of drawing page 98 by Maurice Spira.

The poem *One Day Thesis* was previously published
in The Local and The Coast Reporter, Sechelt, B.C.

Published by Calendula Farms
Box 193 Roberts Creek, B.C. Canada V0N2W0
jcovernton@gmail.com

Fetal Alcohol Spectrum Disorders (FASD) describes a continuum of permanent birth defects caused by maternal consumption of alcohol during pregnancy.
- Wikipedia

"… is it an error, or another point of view?"
- Micheal D. Mann

F.A.S.D. & Me

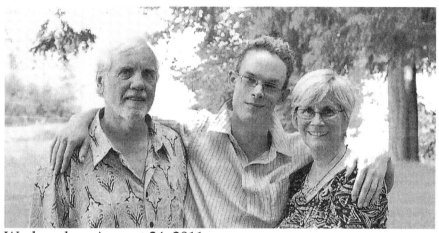

Wednesday, August 24, 2011

Hi. My name is Micheal. I am 29 years of age. I live at home with my long time foster mother and father. I am involved in many activities, have many friends and live a very productive life. In so many ways, I am just like you. One thing though… I have a Developmental Disability. I was born with Fetal Alcohol Spectrum Disorder, or F.A.S.D for short. I have also been diagnosed with Tourette's Syndrome, Asperger's Syndrome (a form of high functioning autism), Obsessive Compulsive Disorder (OCD) and Attention Deficit Hyperactivity Disorder (ADHD).

In my early years, it was difficult for many to understand why I was the way I was. For me however, it was, and is, far more difficult to live the way I am. In my childhood, I encountered numerous challenges, many of which I have overcome, some which still remain in one way or another.

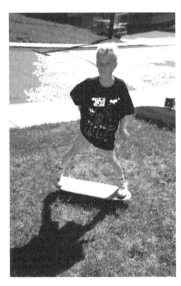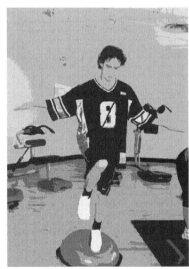

Balance was a huge issue. When I was seven and eight I was still unable to climb the stairs one at a time, for fear of slipping and falling, or in my words "having the ground hit me".

For a long time, walking meant never lifting my feet, only shuffling them on the ground. Now I can run like the wind in Track And Field and have zero fear of falling!

Sensations were something else all together. For example, a time on the beach, walking on rocks with bare feet, I remember being in pain, the unfamiliar feeling of the rocks under my feet. After that I was sure to pack along beach shoes.

The Tourette's began early on as a constant clearing of my throat, graduating to tapping of my feet, to what it is now, which is facial twitching, and constant kneading of my throat in sore or irritated areas.

My doctors and others are now trying to help me with medication and counseling to deal with the OCD, ADHD and my anxiety.

My OCD affects me in ways such as I care VERY much about how I dress, having clothes match, and often over-compensating with hats, jewelry and other knick-knacks.

My ADHD causes me to blank out when I am being told something, and I do try hard to focus, but I seem to only have a slight interest in the topic of conversation. I go everywhere with my iPod, always listening to music. As a matter of fact I am listening to it as I type right now.

Anxiety for me comes when I relate to time, money or other abstract parts of life. I hate to be late, often actively waiting, pacing or mumbling to myself instead of remembering things I have to do to be totally ready.

Money is like this: if I had no controls, I would be broke. This is a part of my OCD and anxiety: have money, will spend, often on nonsense items such as cd's, jewelry or more clothes than I need.

This is the part of the article I am feeling anxious about writing. It is about my social life as a kid. I was *the* target for bullying, simply because of how I reacted to it, namely in a loud and aggressive manner. Bullies learned fast that they could always get me to overreact. No matter what *they* did; my overreaction always got *me* in trouble.

As I grew older, all I wanted was to be accepted and have a group of friends, to be like others I saw around me, with social status, the girls, the money and the popularity. I will talk further about this later.

Reading social cues continues to be an ongoing issue. I may look at someone or see someone and think they are, in a phrase "looking at me the wrong way." Misunderstanding what a person means or says, either from their tone of voice or what they say, often brings conflict as I act on a threat that is only perceived, and not at all reality based.

Having the mouth of a sailor is a BIG problem. Though I show an extensive vocabulary in this article, when I am the least bit irritated or downright raging, expletives are my expression of choice. Social mistakes, using violent words as well as cussing, pushed away the very people I wanted to have close to me, with them becoming increasingly uncomfortable and drifting away.

Waking up to go to school, as far back as elementary was something I dreaded. I had next to no friends, or if I did, I was blind to the fact.

Though there were challenges, I had many gifts that got me through. My ability to do well in English and Social Studies gave me peace of mind. Although I was not popular with the student body, I found solace in the support some of the staff gave me in elementary and secondary schools alike.

As I worked on my gift for the spoken, and especially the written word, I saw a potential that was sure to develop into something much more rewarding in later years. As it turned out, I was more than right.

More often than not I can now articulate how I feel and have it understood. I feel sympathy and have a strong sense of empathy for those I am close to, including friends and family. I am not ashamed to say I cry.

Whether it is a sad song, a sad scene in a movie, feeling lonely, or remembering a past pain, the tears fall steady and true. I also feel the struggle of those I have never met because they are going through what I have endured or they are stuck in a living hell and all I want to do is take them away and make them smile.

My mom reminds me, again and again, that it is important for me to see the love and happiness in each day of my life. When I have a bad day, and conflict ensues, I sink into depression. I have been told to think hard of all the things I am grateful for. I would list them all here but that would be half this article.

I have an extensive interest in music, movies and fashion. I can list off artists, discographies, actors and their many roles, the year an album was released.

I love to dress in good clothes. I often change more than a few times until I feel satisfied with what I have on. As with music and movies, money - a lot of it - goes towards these hobbies.

Finances have been a struggle for me. Only recently, within the past two or three years, have I begun to grasp what it means to have and manage money. Thinking back to the old days, when I was lucky to have five or more dollars in one account, makes me so very grateful for what lies in my two accounts now.

I am currently on PWD – short for Persons With Disabilities. I get a cheque from the Government to help support me financially. Part of the pay goes towards room and board; the rest is divided into two kinds of savings accounts.

Within the past year, Community Living BC has also come to my aid by starting to provide funding for my family and me. This continues to support me and provide money for respite and community inclusion.

Having support around me, to serve as an "external brain" is crucial. Reminders help me to keep track of belongings; a second brain helps me with control and direction. I like that I have my family and respite and mental health workers to listen and offer advice that helps me to stay "on the track" and assist me when I "go off the rails."

As for employment, it's a bit convoluted. I do not have a regular job. I have tried working at a nursery and the SPCA. I have also made several volunteer attempts through a program that offers what can be considered in simple terms as "paid volunteering".

I have what folks call "barriers to employment" that stand in my way. Slowly I am chipping away at these, showing everyone around me that with the right supports, I am learning to manage surprises, changes in plans, and whatever conflicts may arise.

It is a process, and I smile each time with every success. I now have watered plants and continue to vacuum and wash company vehicles for SCACL as well as other odd jobs for an hour and fifteen minutes a week. I smile now, thinking of each job completed as a small success.

In the days of my alcohol and drug use I was drained of money and much more. I started smoking marijuana and drinking alcohol at age 15 and moved on to cocaine and ecstasy and did not stop until 26 years of age. I suffered through a decade plus of addiction.

When I quit, I decided so because I was at a New Years Eve party January 1, 2009 and saw by the end of the night how drugs and alcohol are really a way to spoil a good time and how they can affect the behavior of those around me. By the end of the night I felt unsafe and unhappy, so the next day I came home and said, "That's it, I quit!" I began going to Alcoholics Anonymous meetings and found solace there, a place with folks like me with new sobriety or years of sobriety all supporting themselves and others. I am proud to say now, in 2012 that I am three years clean and sober!

I made what I thought of as "friends" who also drank and used drugs. I was very susceptible and easily influenced, a fancy way of saying I was pretty much a door mat. I had no real social outlets, so unfortunately I went back again and again, looking for something that was never there.

The best way I can sum that up before the next subject of this article is using a famous phrase: "To do the same thing over and over, expecting different results is the definition of insanity". How sadly true.

I have lived many places and in many different environments. To say the least, not all have been conducive to a healthy lifestyle. I have lived in the care of Children's Aid Society, group homes with Mental Health, on the streets, in my own apartment, a motel, and hospital wards and now I am back home. I have had quite a journey.

During those years, Mental Health did not understand how to work with someone like me but with more education from my support network they were able to help me connect with Community Living B.C. I still have a wonderful counselor at Mental Health whose listening skills are amazing and she grants me the gifts of strategies for every day life.

It is hard for others to understand the fact I do have F.A.S.D. and a Developmental Disability, as I am highly functional in many areas, speech, writing and seeking social outlets. Some just assume I am a troublemaker, one who doesn't listen or try hard enough. They think I am "up here" only, not seeing where I am "down here."

To elaborate, having an "invisible disability" makes it difficult for some to see why I can do many things well, but when it comes to losing my temper, or grasping instruction, having tasks being explained many times they think, "Well, Micheal seems like he should understand more than he claims." I tell you this: I wish nothing more than that. I really do.

I am truly grateful for my allies in this life. My mother, father, my many respite and outreach workers, my counselor, coaches and athletes in Special Olympics, and so many others.

Special Olympics has given me the terrific opportunity to take part in sports, something I never could dream of in my school days. I play softball, soccer, basketball, swim and run track & field, and recently dabbled in "floor hockey" of sorts, though the proper term is Ringette. I have learned discipline, skills, pacing and development of patience.

I have attended the gym twice a week, one day partaking in circuit training, the other working with a personal trainer. I feel and see the benefits everyday. I love it.

I have had private swimming lessons to help with my Special Olympics swimming. I love the water. I joke and say it's because I was born a Pisces.

I have also taken and loved horseback riding lessons. When I sit upon the beautiful horses and ride, I feel such a connection, almost like they know how I feel, and more often that not, I see a lot of me in them.

Animals have always been some of my closest friends. Happy, sad, laughing or crying they always know how I'm feeling and are there to support me. I love them all and know they teach me patience, love, trust, loyalty and how to laugh when I am at my lowest.

Writing plays a MAJOR role in how I express myself. Ever since I could pick up a pen or pencil and grab a piece of paper, putting down my emotions, in poetry, song or rhymes, gives me an outlet for all my feelings. I know I would not be the man I am today without it. I have submitted articles and other prose and poetry and had them published. I have performed some of my writing and felt honoured to have people listen.

Each new day carries with it its own list of challenges and tests. Lately I feel I have met these and am overcoming them day-by-day. I know not what lies ahead, today, tomorrow or an hour from now, but I smile knowing I can look any difficulty in the eye and stand up and rise above.

The One-Day Thesis

Good Evening. My name is Micheal and I have a query.

Have you ever felt uneasy
about the man screaming in the street?
about sitting next to the woman talking to herself?
about the teenager with the cuts on her arm?
What if you woke up one day and this was you?
Not an easy thought is it?

Well ladies and gentlemen, welcome to the world of Mental
Illness, FASD or Complex Neurobehavioural Disorders.

We go through our daily lives trying to blend in, fade away,
or exclaim our thoughts.
We want love, friendship, warmth and a sympathetic ear to
listen to our troubles.

We may look or even seem dangerous, nerdy, strange, etc.
But we are as you are - at least we want to be.

We're told to get help, take medication, go to rehab…

Yes, yes, yes. All strong and valid points.

However, we are also looking for a guiding hand to help us and someone to smile back when we smile.

We don't want to be coddled. We just want to be like you.

Thanks for listening.

Mike vs MANN

Life's Rough
> *"I don't give a fuck"*

Not afraid to cry
> *"Hurt me & die"*

Now you can think clearly
> *"Gimmie coke, e, dope n beer"*

Keep your head up, eyes on the prize
> *"Head down, eyes on your enemies"*

2 Sides

1 Man

One U know 'n like

The other with anger 'n hate

Mike vs Mann

Sometimes I don't know who I am

I love those who love me
> *"Can't trust no one, they gon' cross me"*

Can't wait 4 the sun 2 rise
> *"Happy in the dark of night"*

Another day, another opportunity

"I have to open my eyes… shit another day"

Leave the past behind

"Those were the best times"

2 Sides

1 Man

One U know 'n like

The other with anger 'n hate

Mike vs Mann

Sometimes I don't know who I am

Violence only begets more

"Why should my enemy have a chance anymore?"

Smile, laugh, love, live

"Frown, scream, hate and live evil."

Got all the time in the world

"Fuck waiting, been thru' 'nuff I want it all"

No "I" in team

"I'm my own man need no one 2 care 4 me"

2 Sides

1 Man

One U know 'n like

The other with anger 'n hate

Mike vs Mann

Sometimes I don't know who I am

Feed the wolf with the pale coat

"All I see is a pale horse"

Treasure your gifts

"No one gives a shit"

Hey Mann

"Yeah what is it?"

I can't understand

"Understand what?"

Why we are the same person, but so out of touch

"I'm your pain, anger 'n rage"

I'm nice. I've healed. I'm not in a cage

"But U still me, don't ignore me"

Chill with you 2 long be the end of me eventually

"I can see U wanna shed tears, c'mere let me deal with the pain"

I'm a man who cries for that I feel pride

Listen dude don't want to argue

Mann all I'm sayin' is let me hold you

You're 6 years old, soul's so cold

"All I wanted was love and to feel it too"

You can love me and I love you too

2 Sides

1 Man

One U know 'n like

One who sees the light

Mike is that Mann who knows who I am.

Written Wednesday, April 20th, 2011

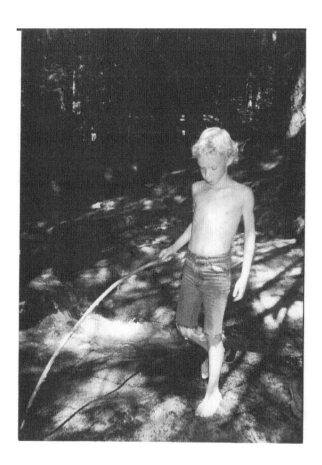

WHITE

I am white.

I feel more wrong than right

The sight in the mirror

Lies inside the evil of the overseer

I realize I am not Islamic, Black,

Jewish, Asian, Hispanic, or First Nations.

All that the world is built on

The backs of non-Caucasians

Sins of the cracker honky wonder bread

Please look at what I said

Know I feel hatred for Bush

Hitler Grand Dragons Nazis of the neo

I see what's real

Canadians fooling ourselves

While sweeping our secrets away, our secrets

Like so many maple leaves

Mr. Suzuki I apologize

For those who won't

Amaru and Abdu, Rodney King,

Geneva Six, I apologize

Realize that the skin of porcelain

The white "Man"

It makes me sad so many understand not

Full meal pots

While others struggle for bread

Behind bars at 16 just because OUR laws were broken

Cocaine creates pain, US who fly the planes

To gather dough we can mold into jaded addicted souls

See not right "not white" crosswalk the street

PD A-R-M-Y Abu G-h-r-a-i-b war for peace

Liquor and Tobacco W(hit)E taxed legal poisons

(mis)informed conscious decisions

I am not afraid at all to say

I'm white and this I hate.

Working With F.A.S.D.

Living

Loving

Dealing

A lot of people are trained how to work with children, teens, as well as adults who live each day with passion over adversity.

People like me need the help of these understanding and trustworthy individuals to guide and to be there when any challenge should arise.

The challenges include:

1. Organization,

2. Social interaction, i.e., cues,

3. Handling finances,

4. Household work, such as cooking or cleaning or yard work,

5. Sports.

Now to people who are not a hundred percent sure how to approach someone with fetal alcohol spectrum disorder, here are a few tips.

Always know that no matter how bad the situation looks the client will get over it. He or she will most likely feel remorse for any negative behaviour that could have been, or was, disruptive and/or destructive.

Have a plan set out (I call mine a Situations and Techniques or S.A.T. plan), that the client can refer to with his or her worker to go over feelings, reasons for feelings, and solutions for problems. This plan describes feelings, reactions, and alternative behaviours and lays out how situations transpired.

Respite workers are also essential, especially for the parents of a child, teen or adult with Fetal Alcohol Spectrum Disorder; a place where the client can go to relax and give the caregivers or parents some time to get back to their own lives.

Having open conversations between counselors, psychologists, and psychiatrists as it pertains to the parents is very important. This way everyone is "in the loop" and everybody can discuss the best way to support the client.

Encouraging talents of a client with disabilities is so important. Whether they paint, sing, build, or write, focus on their special abilities and you will see a spark that will light the sky. I promise you this.

I hope with these few points you now have an understanding that will make it easier to live, care for and love us who have a special place here on the great world.

Just because we are disabled does not mean we don't have abilities to bring a smile to anyone's face.

Thanks.

On Horseback

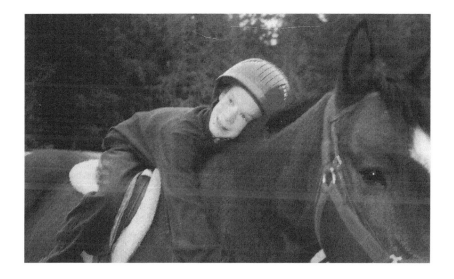

The horseback riding I participate in is called *therapeutic riding.* For folks like me, either with developmental disabilities or those with even more severe impairments, therapeutic riding allows for one-on-one care with the instructor and student to improve skills such as balance, coordination, listening skills, and even frustration issues. I love this form of riding and encourage anyone with a child or client who has a disability to enroll them in a class. I can predict you will see great changes in behavior, as well as ability, in a short amount of time.

I began riding horses at the age of ten. I don't have a clear memory of that early experience. What does strike me is how vivid my time was with Susan Milne, and Comet and Harley. I remember learning so much from Susan at her stables on Crowe Road. I learned how to trot, to steer and how to quicken a horse's step. I believe I even cantered once or twice!!

What I really mean to say is when I am riding a horse whether it was Comet or Harley, or more recently Tivio or Patches, there is an unspoken connection between the horse and me as the rider. This connection is felt as far down as my very soul.

Comet was the first horse that Susan Milne had me ride. Comet was an older horse, and eventually he grew too old, and me too big, so onto Harley I rode. Now Comet was a funny horse, old and set in his ways, and liked to pull fast ones. Susan and I shared plenty of laughs while I rode him. Harley, a younger, stronger horse, was even more of a trickster. He figured he'd show *me* who was boss. Many times I had to correct him, but eventually we were both on the same page.

Susan Milne is a lady, very sweet, calm, stern, but gentle and always loved to see the horses and me working together. I learned plenty from her way of teaching, repetitive, reassuring and always with care. I miss my times with Susan, and still run into her around the Coast. She smiles fondly when she tells me of a photo she has of me on Harley in her tack room.

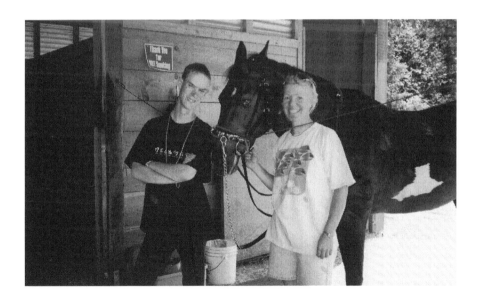

Tivio was the first horse that I rode when I began my lessons with Tracy Gray. Tivio was FULL of tricks and LOVED to take control when he could, cutting corners, stopping mid-trot, cutting in too close to Tracy etc. But when he listened, Tivio and I were like water, always in fluid motion as one.

The newest horse I ride, Patches, does incredibly well despite having cataracts in his left eye, which sometimes cause him to work more on his right side; a minor thing of course. He likes to test me sometimes as well, seeing how far he can go before I tell him otherwise. With him I feel a special connection as I have accomplished so much while riding him, including learning the different spots around the ring such as "riding large" which is riding along the rail and how to steer him using only my feet and legs and almost no reins. Yay for me!

Tracy Gray is truly a great teacher. Kind and encouraging, sweet and all the wonderful things that remind me so much of Susan Milne. With these two women I have been given a great gift. Thanks go out to both women.

Horses are very sensitive creatures. One must always be of sound mind and body before attempting a ride. Just as your best friend can feel what you do, so can the horse. So away let your troubles go before you swing that leg over and stirrup your feet.

Being calm in your ride you can still feel the emotions, sadness, frustration etc. but if you are sound, I have found it is highly therapeutic to be on horseback. Picture a time at the counselor's office. There is where you can explain all your troubles in a safe environment right? It is the same on the horse. The horse can feel your pain and, through you gently riding, can soothe you and allow you to go through what you are feeling with amazing grace.

The feelings of accomplishment I have felt, as I'm sure many others have too, are astounding. From the first correct steering, to the finish of a two-point stance, each step in technique achieved gives me a feeling of "WOW!"

I would like to take this time to honor Susan Milne and Tracy Gray for all their hard work and dedication to me and first and foremost to the horses in their care. You both have taught me so much about being myself and believing in myself. For that I thank you both so very much.

To all the horses I have ridden in my time of therapeutic riding I want to give a big *HUG* and a soft pat. You have done so much for me and continue to do so. God bless you wonderful creatures.

Stand Up Paddle Boarding

'SUP? I want to tell you about my experience with Stand Up Paddle Boarding.

Stand Up Paddle Boarding, or SUP'ing, or in the language of the Hawaiian people **Hoe he'e nalu,** is a sport that originated in Hawaii in the 1960's. The beach boys of Waikiki, a neighbourhood in Honolulu, would paddle out on long boards to watch over the people surfing. This gave it another nickname "Beach Boy Surfing".

I had this experience for the first time in Halfmoon Bay, right here on our beautiful Sunshine Coast.

I was apprehensive but also very excited to undertake this new challenge. Would I be able to maintain my balance? Could I stay on the board for more than 2 minutes?

At first, and for a while, I only sat on or lay down on the paddleboard using my hands and/or the paddle.

Then once I had done that for long enough I thought to myself, "Okay Mike, they call it a STAND UP paddleboard for a reason." So up I got and, boy, when I had my first fall it was a doozy!

Walked backwards right off the board! I laughed so hard I wish someone had gotten it on film. It was straight out of the cartoons!

Eventually I gained enough balance by just simply looking ahead and avoiding looking down, as that would quickly disorient me. I got to a point when all of a sudden I was paddling with, get this, my eyes closed! I didn't fall either! I was so proud and amazed at my feat.

It was fun and lots of it. My thanks to Paula Bowie for introducing me to this fabulous sport. Stand Up Paddle Boarding is definitely on my list of activities for future summers.

Saturday, December 17, 2011

A SPECIAL OLYMPIC
4 SYLLABLE VERSE

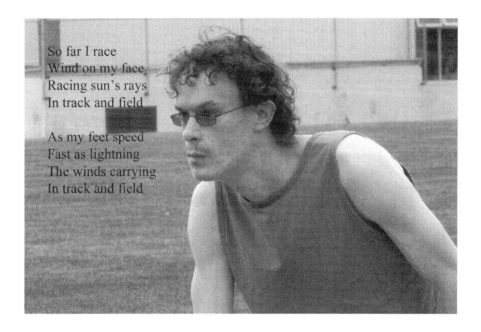

So far I race
Wind on my face
Racing sun's rays
In track and field

As my feet speed
Fast as lightning
The winds carrying
In track and field

Throw metal ball

Give it your all

Measure when fall

In track and field

Run and you jump

Land with a clump

Try to stand up

In track and field

Dribble the ball

Careful don't fall

Stand proud and tall

Play basketball

Bounce and chest pass

Don't you talk trash

Try to not to crash

Play basketball

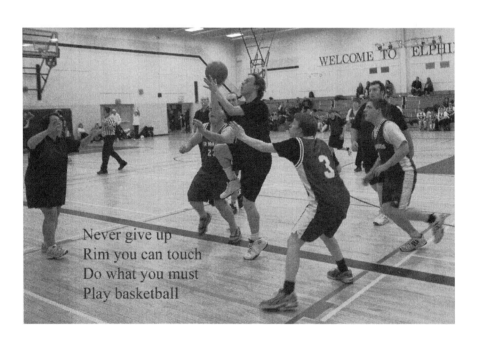

Never give up
Rim you can touch
Do what you must
Play basketball

No board at all
Swish all the ball
Net catches all
Play basketball

Using your feet
It's pretty neat
To score a feat
Playing soccer

Up and down grass
Really quite fast
Pride is a badge
Playing soccer

Green black and white
All colors bright
Kick from the side
Playing soccer

Hit a homerun
Round bases run
It's so much fun
Playing softball

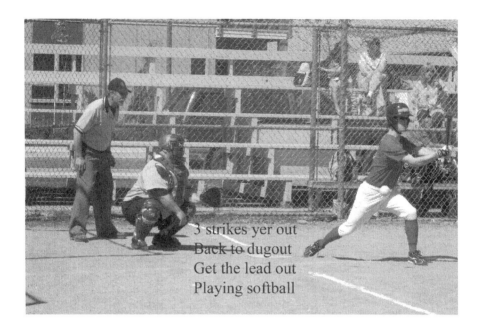

3 strikes yer out
Back to dugout
Get the lead out
Playing softball

Victory's shown

Best beaten own

Nice you condone

Playing softball

Deep in you dive

Move with such drive

Best of your time

When you're swimming

Front stroke and back

Breaststroke and kick

Adults or kids

When you're swimming

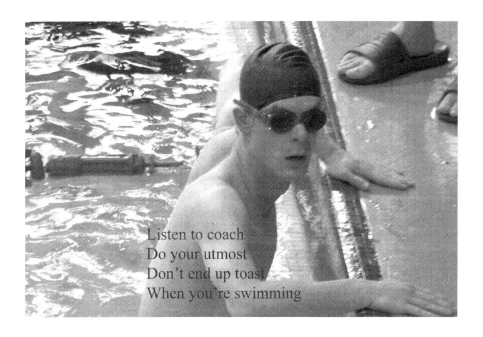

Listen to coach
Do your utmost
Don't end up toast
When you're swimming

Friends they are made

Games they are played

Memories made

When we compete

Memories kept

Ready get set

You're dry or you're wet

When we compete

In Special O

Watch us all go

The Player's Oath

When we compete:

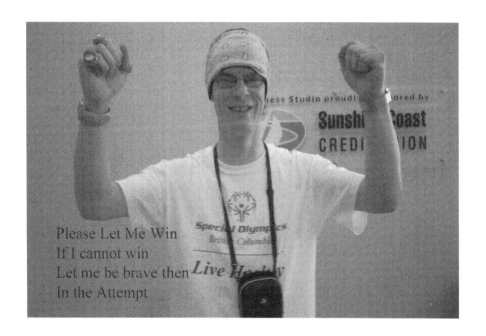

Challenges I Face

Every day I wake up looking forward to another day. I don't however look forward to the problems I encounter every morning, noon and night.

Whether I'm in a situation I do not understand, stuck in a conflict, trying my best to focus when distracted or feeling anxious, so many problems can arise.

I may lose my temper, resorting to cussing and childlike behaviour such as kicking and punching walls and stomping my feet. When I am approached by people who seek to calm me, I lash out at them, in my words "seeing red." I wind up losing support at a time when I need it the most. Though I may at that time seek help and forgiveness, I fret that not all are ready to give it freely.

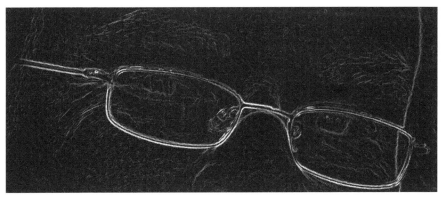

Anger, I know is a secondary emotion. I may be feeling many different emotions at a time. That for me is overwhelming, and results in loss of composure and leaves me in the wake of a blow up. After a blow up, I feel horrible. Embarrassed does not even begin to cover it. I look at who may be around after I lose it, and automatically want to crawl in a hole and never come out. I have lost my temper and exploded in restaurants, grocery stores, in the middle of the street, you name it. I am sure many folks have a mental image of me going ballistic somewhere here on the Sunshine Coast where I live. Triggers can be many things. One in particular is when I run into people from my past who are troublemakers and I end up in a confrontation, which leaves me in a rage because they have pushed my buttons.

The fact I choose anger as the primary emotion to show only makes life harder.

Other challenges rear their heads often: money management, time management, and staying on task or doing something that is challenging for the first time.

Making the best of a waiting period is not exactly a strong point for me either. If I have an event in a day that takes place at noon, I am dressed and "ready to go" at 8 in the AM. Sounds crazy right? Well it's a reality for me. Active waiting and pacing instead of being productive around the house is a well-practiced fallback position for me.

Money is the root of a lot of arguments about "independence". I use quotations because I know perfectly well I need an external brain and secondary judgment when it comes to finances, otherwise I would not be in the fortunate financial situation I currently find myself enjoying. If it was up to my lack of good decisive action, I would be broke. No joke.

When I am working outside, doing yard work or garage organization, I lose stamina very quickly, as well as focus, and drive to finish the task at hand, wanting to be inside on my computer or watching television rather than contributing my help to whatever task is at hand.

Needless to say, it is not necessarily easy nor hard being me, just a day at a time does the trick. As long as I remember techniques given to me to focus and maintain my temper when I am triggered, whether by conflict, a sudden change in plans, or something lost or misplaced, I am, more often than not, now smoothing myself out before anything major takes place. I am proud of that. I really am.

Couplet of a Bad Day

One day I had an unfortunate start,
angry tone arose in my heart.
Off Dad and I went to recycling,
and came fast bad troubles cycling.
Reminders of things well known
allowed for annoyance and ignorance shown;
eyes were rolled
at all, words told.

Came to gym though for a while
took less than that to behave as child:
challenged by stranger unfamiliar
he became target of pent-up anger.
Off went glasses and out-of-way machine.
I yelled, I cussed, I yelled I screamed.
Even after removal from that place
angry body language took their place.
Drove home in angry state,
growled as I began to contemplate

long talk with papa and ma, a fuss
to mediate what divided us.

Today I pick myself back up
and only wish for better luck.

Note: in writing practice I have been using the book *In Fine
Form* by Kate Braid and Sandy Shreve (Polestar, 2005) to
explore writing in different poetic forms. I have worked on
couplets, haiku, and sonnets, among others.

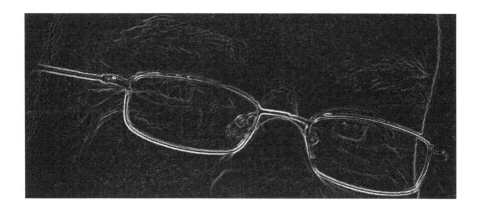

A Punch In The Face (a story)

The sun beat down on the cool concrete in the late afternoon at a bus stop on Cowichan Street. A man stood there, earphones blasting Bob Seger's "Turn The Page" from his Sony MP3 player. Mark had just gotten off work at the Suncoast Wine and Bottle. He had done an excellent job at washing a company vehicle as well as tidying up the office. It was small labour but it was a job and Mark was happy to have it.

Along came one of Mark's old acquaintances, Harold. Mark and Harold had done some pretty crazy things back in Mark's younger days, and since then, he had not seen Harold for quite a while.

"Hey Harold," said Mark, "How's it going?"

"Not bad," replied Harold, "Just finished a meeting at the local Community Support Office."

"How did that go?" Mark asked.

"Well, I was able to receive some funds for my household bills."

"Excellent."

Now, coming up the street was a younger acquaintance of Mark's. This young man, Terry, was not in the same mood as Harold or Mark. Terry stumbled up to them.

"Dude, I just got into it with a couple of guys, you should've seen it! It was wicked!"

Now Mark and Terry had had their share of crazy times together as well. Let's just say they were known to knock back more than a few in the old days. Mark could smell the scent of Olde English 800 on Terry's breath.

Mark replied to Terry's boasting by playfully smacking the back of Terry's head.

Did he know what would happen next?

SMACK

Mark held his face where Terry's fist had met it, along the left side of his jaw.

"Don't try that again dude," said Terry.

Mark was feeling so many things at this one moment. Angry. Shocked. Fearful. Betrayed.

He calmly said to the air "Excuse me, just give me a second here."

He went into the local delicatessen took out his cellphone and quickly dialed the local police dispatch.

"911 Emergency, fire, ambulance or police?" came a soft female voice over the speaker.

"Police please" replied Mark.

A moment passed and by then, Mark had walked back out to the bus stop, seeing no sign of either Harold or Terry.

"Police, what is the matter?" came another woman's voice over the cell phone.

"Yes, my name is Mark Datsun and I have just been physically assaulted, I request police to apprehend Terry Ortiz immediately."

"Okay, and what is your location sir?" came the voice again, sweet sounding, calm and reassuring.

"I am standing at a bus stop on Cowichan Street, across the road from The Bank Of Royals."

"What is Mr. Ortiz wearing Mark?"

At this time, Mark was growing quite weary of the questions, and without thinking let the woman on the line know just that. "Look, find the jerk or I will, got it?" he exclaimed.

"Please sir, remain calm, I am only trying to help you here ok?" the woman replied "Now what was Mr. Ortiz wearing?"

"A beige hoodie and an army fatigue design baseball cap."

"And how tall is he?"

Mark thought about this for a minute.

He was hazy on this fact but he figured Terry must be at least his size, Mark being dang near 5'8, and Terry being at least 5'6.

"5 Feet 6 inches." Mark replied.

"Ok and where is he now?"

"He took off through the alley adjacent to the Bank Of Royals, heading east towards Spear Point Apartments."

"Ok, an officer should be on his wa…"

Just then a cruiser passed by and Mark waved it down. He could hear the dispatchers voice over the cruiser's radio and knew he had found someone to talk to.

"Are you Mark Datsun?" asked the officer.

"Yes sir I am"

The officer repeated some of the questions the dispatcher had relayed to him, and so Mark gave the same answers, this time biting his tongue, as not to repeat the previous threat spoken to the dispatcher.

Just then the 2:45 bus to Bobby's Lake arrived, and Mark did not want to miss it.

"My cell phone number is 064-899-0043, please call me when you have a chance. It's a must I catch this bus."

"Will do sir," replied the officer.

With that said and done, Mark got on the bus for home to eat dinner and prepare for his BBall practice that night, which he looked forward to immensely.

EPILOGUE

Mark arrived, ate dinner, and went to his basketball practice. He did not speak of the incident again until later that evening when Officer Henderson came by to visit.

"Now Mark," began Officer Henderson "You do understand the seriousness of what you said to our dispatch, don't you?"

"When I said find Terry or else, right?" replied Mark.

"Yes, now I understand the heat of the moment, but you have to understand that on my way here I was having a bit of trouble figuring out what to do, whether I should arrest you for uttering threats or not."

"I am sorry for my outburst, officer," Mark replied.

"I know that, so I have come the conclusion that I will not bring you in, however I cannot bring Terry in either. I can warn him to stay away from you or he will be charged with assault. Is that ok?"

"I see no problem with that sir."

"Good then, well I best be on my way."

"I see now, that in a situation where someone is inebriated it's best NOT to engage them in ANY way, Officer Henderson. It only leads to hassle. Thanks for stopping by."

In the weeks after, Mark got over his problems with Terry and continued on with his life. All was well.

What Is Writing to Me?

Writing has always been something I have turned to with more of a whim than with an actual purpose. Loose-leaf pages are piled high in disarray. Poems, hip hop rhymes, some of which are either introspective or just plain old "what I feel like writing about."

I have only now, within this year and a half, begun to truly understand what it means to write.

Though I have begun and finished several published works and performed a few as well, the art of writing really stays with me as a tool of my love for the way words can be put together to clear my head, put a "dope rhyme" together or grab paper and pen and just do it!

Music really started, and still highly influences, my words when I write. I mentioned previously about hip-hop. In my early teens I discovered this genre of music and, in my eyes (and ears), I saw and heard the anger I felt as a teen that was different.

I have to admit, sheepishly, I do not keep a steady journal, nor do I write everyday. I see myself as somewhat of a writer, but truth be known, I only really write when I feel inspired at the time.

(When I wrote this in 2010 it was true but now I have a daily writing practice.)

They say to truly undertake a profession or a title is to be 100% dedicated. One's art must come before anything frivolous. I know I must "get off my ass" and get to task. I can say I'm writing something, but really if it is half done, and does not pick up for a long time, I am not "writing" I am "speaking."

I do know that I am merely quoting advice given to me, and I need to hammer it into my brain.

I write well and I can write better.

I am very happy to have this chance to learn to push myself and ascertain whether I can be the kind of wordsmith I see myself as in my head.

I say this not to put myself down or to criticize myself, only to say what I already know. I love to write, and I know writing loves me. However, as in any relationship, the effort has to be balanced fairly on each end.

In closing, I would like to acknowledge some of my inspirations for my love of the written word….

Tupac Amaru Shakur
Stephen King
Ron Braunstein
Tim McGraw

Marshall Mathers

Bob Dylan

All the times of anger, love, sadness, grief and joy in what is known as life.

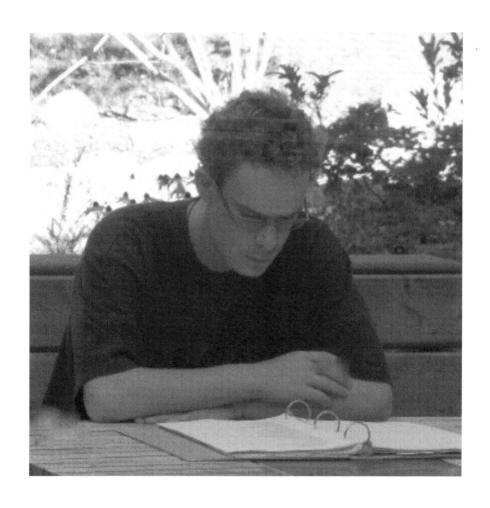

Whatever Happened?

Whatever happened to a teenager helping a senior citizen across the street? Or seeing a homeless person on the street, buying them a hot meal, and paying for their stay in a warm bed?

I'll tell you people.

Those are the ideals of a better world that have somehow become drowned by the build up of McDonald's triple low fat lattes, Gucci, and the latest Hollywood blockbuster.

I am saying this as a person not only on the outside of this spectrum but inside of it as well. The old adage goes "Stand for something or fall for anything." I have fallen many times but I am looking for an answer and when I saw nothing but sex, crime, and the fast dollar idolized, my eyes shone with what I knew were empty stars.

So many people hold on to their pain and let it build. Another adage that I believe not to be so true now is "Grown men don't cry." We all cry.

War. Famine. Children becoming orphans in infancy - Why? I ask this because I know that if all of us, including me, really thought about it, we could do something to bring it to an end.

The next time a "pro" asks you "looking for a good time?" buy her new clothes and take her to a clinic and pay for a rest in a reputable hotel and food as well, so she can be healthy, warm, fed and safe from those who would use her and do her harm.

If you know of a drug dealer in your neighborhood get him off the street and in jail to keep his rat poison off the streets and away from innocents.

If you notice a child hanging in the wrong crowd, alert a local youth center and his parents, giving that young person a chance to grow up and find the cure for cancer or run the next 100-mile marathon.

If nothing else, change the most important thing in the world…

You.

Monday, December 5, 2011

I Am a Man Who Cries

Tears fall from my eyes
The world has so much suffering and pain
It's so insane
I want to save
Release all from the cage
Fly the skies
Open their eyes
No hate
No need to fight
Make wrong right
Because every earth's entity has
The universal right
To celebrate existence
To the utmost delight.
Remove soldiers from their posts
Take them where they're needed most
Into the arms of their children and wives
Poor children on the corner
Nothing but the clothes on their back
And fear in their eyes
Why?! Am I allowed to be happy
When they are not?!
So wrong that so many are blind
Free them from the shackles
That bind.
Let them see the smiles
In their parent's eyes
A warm bed
Good food

The loser shall win
No woman shall cringe from a man
Stand tall make that tyrant fall
Everyone shall march no longer crawl
Please heed this call
I cry for her him them us
I cry from all the pain
I want all of it to fade
Tears fall from my eyes
I am a man who cries.

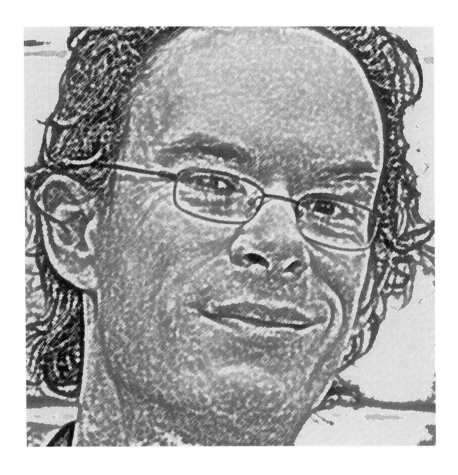

Journal Writing

Today I feel a lot of things. Frustrated, bored, lonely, ticked off, excited, worried, anxious, happy, sad and in love.

I feel these things because I have a girlfriend who I rarely spend ANY time with. I am wondering and worrying about our future as a couple if we don't have any time spent together. By the way I am amazed right now that I am NOT looking at the keyboard right now as I type this. My fingers just seem to be able to find the keys. I am in a zone.

As I was saying about my girlfriend, I do love her, but I feel frustrated and lonely that we hardly have any time together as a couple to explore each other's personalities, quirks and quarks, and what makes each other tick, so we can be sure that we are actually compatible. I am anxious that I will allow my frustration to be a contributing factor to bad behavior such as snapping at my parents, being angry, with misplaced feelings of being fed up with spending next to no time with her other than on internet chat or on the phone.

I don't want to blow the whole day just because I am in the dumps and wanting to stay and wallow in "why me?"

I had a problem at church yesterday. I felt the sermon touched on something that really hits a nerve with me. The Minister said that one has a *choice* to believe in a different God other than mine, but that the person is *wrong*. This I abhor. I feel as a good Christian I cannot go about judging another person's beliefs. I am being a judge about that person and I have no right if I want to be what the Christian faith embraces, love and acceptance for all.

I am excited about going out later for lunch at Tim Hortons and spending my gift cards I got for Christmas. I might even hang out with M, a younger bud of mine, who by the way is funny as heck. I smile right now thinking of me and him goofing around.

I have to write for an hour. I guess I can just type out my thoughts here as they come. Or maybe I'll write some couplets and haikus, or some free form poetry, or a rap, or another type of song. I don't know yet.

I DO NOT KNOW YET

WHAT I WILL DO FOR MY WORK

THOUGHTS BLOCKED LIKE BEAVER DAM.

(A HAIKU FOR YOU!)

JOURNAL ENTRY FOR TODAY
Thursday, February 9, 2012

Today I will arrive at work at approximately 1:30 pm and finish at 2:30 pm. I am looking forward to seeing everyone there and doing what I do best which is washing or vacuuming the blue or gold van, taking out trash, re-bagging the cans and sweeping the office.

I am writing this journal entry to fill my quota of writing time for one hour. I started at 10:15 am this morning and will finish around 11:15 am or later. I enjoy writing a journal entry because it allows me to express feelings about the day and such. I hope today is a great day without ANY problems. I look forward to work and hope I have NO bad experiences with anyone. I will apologize to the woman for my rudeness at the pool yesterday.

I also am looking forward to going to basketball tonight and being a good sport and not being a dick to those around me. It's just a practice and a scrimmage. I'm not in the frigging NBA or anything.

I want to get out the door in one piece with NO arguments between my folks and I. That would be terrific. I like when I can look back on a day and say "Wow, what an awesome day front to back" It makes me feel great.

I can't wait till this Saturday because I am going to Vancouver AGAIN for a Healthy Athletes event. I will be going with x and I know she will benefit greatly.

I called her last night to wish her sweet dreams and called her this morning to wish her a good day. I will do so for a while I think, just to be a good boyfriend.

I gotta go, my laptop's waiting! Honey Nut, Multi Grain, Frosted, Chocolate Cheerio!!

Monday, February 20, 2012

FEELINGS I HAVE HAD

I sit here feeling the pain of others. Orphaned children, abused mothers, fathers locked up unjustly cuz they were unlucky to be in the system that is designed to enslave them…

I sit here feeling the rage of those trapped in a cage of circumstance. A life of tension and frustration, left homeless from gentrification. If I ain't spelled that word right it's cuz I don't live that alright? With me saying that, I feel like shat shit I mean sitting in a cell without a trace of a gleam of sunlight just cuz you were trying your best to put food on your family's table at night…

I sit here feeling sick of being fortunate, feeling sick that I feel like a hypocrite, with children as young as five digging in trash bins for food just to survive. I'm typing this on a computer, while a man who is sent to a war he don't want to be in, writing a letter to his wife pregnant with his baby girl on a muddy rain soaked three line notepad…

I'm listening to songs about truth, truth I know, some from seeing or feeling, or truth I know nothing about absolutely…

Here is my pain for this electronic page…Born to a mother who loved me willingly, but the cruel hand that life played took me away so many times from a baby to that final time at six years of age. I still remember that face, black eyes, black hair, black beard the way the strikes would make my flesh sear and the constant tears. Going through life not knowing what made me different till I found out my life had been tinted, no tainted by alcohol, fetal alcohol syndrome, foster home after home, found the one that worked, but still I was found again by my hunting curse, left at early teens, with the lies of my closed eyes, thought the world held more, little did I know how much more, went from the only home I'd known back to the one I once thought I knew, came back as an adult even more fucked up, ups and downs thru my 20's drugs, alcohol, pills, coke snorted through $10's, drowning my tears in Olde English 40's late nite phone calls to those I love, high and or drunk, soul feeling sunk over promises made sober, later they were cheated on by a jealous lover addiction, went clean once, left again, back with the black widow again… I am no longer there in the cave, but everyday I feel the pain, my pain, her pain, his pain, your pain, their pain, the pain of the world, sending my mind into an emotional turmoil…

Even though I can feel all the other pain, truth is that's a lie, I'm not in a prison cage, I don't live on the street, I don't sell drugs or myself for drugs to take booze to drink or food to eat, it drives me crazy so much wrong in this world, too much for this song...

AIDS, POVERTY, CHILD SLAVERY, RACIAL PROFILING, THOSE FIGHTING OR LIVING IN A WAR TORN COUNTRY, DISCRIMINATION, FALSE DOMINATION, CUZ OF SEXUAL ORIENTATION OR CHOICE OF RELIGION, STRUCK BY THOSE WHO "LOVE" YOU, LOVE WITH NO LOVE, JUST FEAR...

IT HURTS YOU ALL SO MUCH I FEEL TEARS, BUT THESE ARE TEARS OF SYMPATHY, TEARS CUZ I WANT YOU TO BE WHERE I BE, TEARS CUZ I WANT TO BE WHERE U BE HELPING YOU TO BE WHOEVER AND WHEREVER YOU BE...

I FIND SOLACE IN THE NOTES OF MUSIC AND THE STROKES OF THIS KEYBOARD AND I WANT YOU ALL TO KNOW, IF YOU FEEL ALONE, CLOSE YOUR EYES,

SEE MY HAND AND TAKE HOLD...

AS A FRIEND TOLD ME...

"PUT YOUR HAND IN THE HAND"

Reaching Men with my Writing

In my opinion, being a man gives me a reason and strategies to reach men at their core. I believe that not many men (including myself) really know what is going on inside them.

The old saying, "Grown men don't cry" or show little to no emotion outside of anger and pride is very true, and that is unfortunate. When I write my poetry or any prose, I seek to penetrate the armour that many men build up around their hearts and souls, to allow me a glance at what truly makes them who they are.

Now I know that this is not true for all men, and for that I am grateful. Any man who can open himself up and tell me his fears, insecurities, or pain, I am willing to lend an ear.

Being that I am male, I know how it feels on both sides of the proverbial fence. I do hold some things back, but also allow more emotions, positive and negative, than maybe I should. For me to resort to anger in a situation that is confusing or frustrating is a *constant problem*. I do not take the time to sit and figure out the appropriate actions to take; I just simply go with what has been learned and easy. I as a man need to help myself overcome this obstacle.

So when I write a piece such as "I Am A Man Who Cries" I am openly admitting that if the situation calls for it, and I have no other options open to me, I will shed tears in times of frustration, embarrassment, heartbreak, or if I am moved by a written piece, movie scene, or song. I am, at my best, empathetic to how others must be feeling and I respond accordingly.

I wish this for more men, and above all I wish it for me. I need to focus on what makes me a man that most folks would like to have around, one who is caring, loving, thoughtful, and mindful of my behavior and how it affects those around me.

In summation of this piece I would like to thank the men in my life for showing me what they know and sharing many good times with me. I adore you all and look forward to life with you all in it.

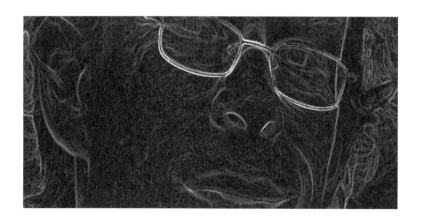

Poetry

My early poetry (age 20 to 25) was written during my days as an alcohol and drug user. That's the reason you may find it dark and somewhat morbid and self-seeking, as during this time I was quite lost and looking for a way out.

My other poems focus on life's questions and follies, love, friendship, and seeking to find my own voice.

I am sure you will love my earlier work (ages 8 to 12) as it was sweeter and less complicated.

So much of my work has been inspired by music. My apologies if I have inadvertently "stolen" an idea. It was out of love.

I am happy you are about to read my poems and to get to know me a little better.

Micheal D.Mann

The Sun of Love

Love is like the sun.
It isn't always there.
I wish it would last longer
so we could be together.

Chorus
Love is like the sun
If you expected it to be there.
Sometimes love is like the clouds
It doesn't act very nicely

Relationships don't last too long
I sure wish they would.
Love is like a donut.
It's there
Then it's gone

Love is sometimes like the sweet thing
Of my life
Sometimes love is like a thunderstorm
It is the worst thing of my life.

La-La-la-la-la

The End

May 1990 (age 8)

Deep appreciation to Laurie Kyle for really listening to my songs and then writing down this, my first piece ever.

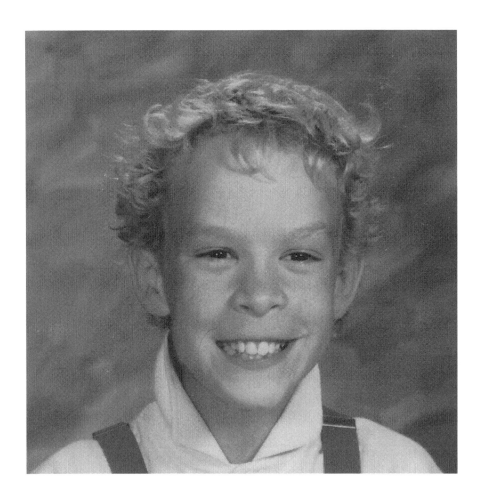

Platinum

Music playing
Thoughts racing
Talking to my teddy bear

My teddy bear
Furry and funny
Warm and loving
Eyes that make me
Grin and laugh away
Doubts that plague me

When I cry
I clutch him tight
Lyin' somber thru the night

When dawn stabs darkness
With the days' waking light
I look at teddy
And I feel all right.

Love you Platinum!

1994

Sunday Rain

As I sit on the window ledge watching life pass me by

Streaks of rain run down the window.

Funny, was not the sun just shining a moment ago?

I look but alas I cannot see as clearly as before

Sunday rain

Sunday rain

Falling down on the holy cross of the church as people come

to pray and to confess their evil sins

Sunday rain

Sunday rain

Falling down on the people too busy making money to notice

the perils surrounding them

Not seeing the others who are working just to keep a home

Whether it be a doorway

Or a cardboard villa

And still others with nothing but their hearts and souls

Who have no one else to share their love

Sunday rain

Sunday rain

Refresh not only nature but us as well

Us with our weapons, drugs and ignorance

Help us Sunday rain

Dear God, wipe your tears

Help us Sunday rain

Oh please be there when needed

Sunday rain.

(About 1994)

Descriptive Essay On Human Subject

She is a natural beauty, with flowing dark hair and fair skin soft as satin. Any man could drown in her deep brown eyes that twinkle with just a hint of wickedness. Her smile turns night to day, winter to summer and fall to spring.

Her personality is that of a girl caught between being a woman yet still a girl. She is bright and intelligent and sweet with a sense of humor that could make Michaelangelo's David crack a smile. She is innocent but in no way naïve, she stands somewhere between the courage of Joan Of Arc and the seductiveness of Lolita.

She is up on stage, dressed in performer's garb, reciting her lines like a true professional, with a voice that cannot be equaled or rivaled by even a robin's sweetest song. She is slightly nervous; she keeps her cool though, showing confidence matching Glen Close in Hamlet. Her radiance is brighter than the sun in the Arctic.

This girl or shall I say young woman, embodies everything that is great and pure of females. Strong willed, beautiful and talented, I wish her only the best in the life ahead of her.

(2002 Pathfinders Essay)

Thank you to Pat Thompson and Rick Bishop for encouraging me to write while I was attending Pathfinders Alternate School.

Bloody Ink

This life got me clutching my Virgin Mary medal.

So much sinning, tear drops, death pains, man I ain't kidding.

What I'm saying is that I'm scared of incarceration.

As a young man wilding, stressing, leading to weed smoking.

One fifty-one guzzling to drown out

Don't know what I'd do without my

homies by my side who can I trust truly?

Snake meat a daily delicacy.

A smile on the face equal to a knife in the back.

Best back up before I react.

Swing a bat with the strength of Thor's hammer.

Feel my power tremour when I spit my facts.

Much more than a simple rap an intricate glance

into my soul trying ever so hard to keep my cool.

A thug's heart beats in my chest every day I test.

Will I ever make it through?

If I love you, trust me.

If I hate you, beware of the eventual pain so insane.

Strapped with the pride of a soldier my instinct my

consigliore ever so wary.

I carry myself like a don grabbing the glock

off the shelf "releasing my delf"* like blood through ink on this page.

A glimpse into a man controlled by rage hitting like a hollow tip to your third eye.

Please just try.

Me.

See what I'm saying you bow down no playing.

What do you think?

Drink bloody ink and you can match me.

August 2006

Method Man, Tical, 1994

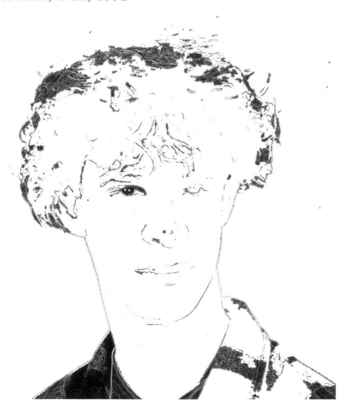

No One

What lies ahead for a soul like me?

Who to trust?

Who's my enemy?

Close friends I confide in

Can I escape sin?

Before I was 6, knew too

much about sex

And how one bled.

Innocence corrupted

Love and trust interrupted.

Trouble sleeping

Flashbacks creeping

Menacingly.

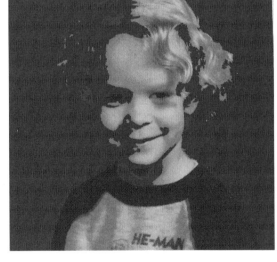

Standing tall,

But I want to fall

Back on my knees

Begging the Goddess to take me away

From my tears,

My fears

My feelings of insecurity

Pondering my exact place in society.

Why am I here?

So much hate, but I want to love.

I know people love,

- me?

Suspicions of what they might have against

Feeling nothing but angst.

Paranoid? Yes.

Stress unbelievable,

Smoking on residual

Just to feel tranquil.

Always with the moon, never in the sun,

Feel like I have no one.

2007

a poem I wrote today

Struggle

What lies behind words

Pride

Wanting what is best

But for whom I ask?

Me who wants to have it all?

Or those I cherish

Those I have regretfully stepped upon to my understanding

now perhaps?

So many turns in this road but somehow I stay in the

roundabout

I feel comfort in this unfortunate numbness

Cold once to all outside

Feeling the flame of change

Burning away all I know

But does it reveal what once was known?

Harsh spoken to love

Anger stricken to caring

Tears equal pride

Make it go away so I can feel strong again

Feel number one

Gaze at my reflection

Quilt design

So many faces

It's as if my own ego self has shattered the glass

"Everything is fine"

"I'm ok"

"No I can handle it"

False yet prophetic words

Uttered as almost a mantra

The key to the lock of my own ignorance

Keeping me caged in my liquor cabinet

My cannabis humidor

Chains placed ever so lovingly

By hands of own

Around outside existence

Out the door

Office

Family

Friendship

Will I win this torturous endeavour?

I see maybe not

Or with a deep breath,

perhaps.

November 23, 2007

When I Die

When I die will I fly?

I see the world thru eyes

That have witnessed evil

Life so vile it seemed unreal

Abused child to a teen livin' wild

Breakin' the law feeling hate for all

That I have been presented

Rememberin' back to no parental presence

Stepdad drunken

Me and Mom sufferin'

Indescribable beatings

Fast forward to criminal meetings

Smokin' and drinkin'

Plotting and schemin'

Hurting and stealin'

Will I pay tithes and do penance for my transgressions?

I see crows wishing they were doves

Wonder will I ever meet the woman that I'll love?

Peace is unbeknownst

Seeking condolence

From a joint or a bottle of beer

To feel brave

Body cold from fear

Life's not all that is perceived

Beware of what you might believe

Sometimes I ponder

When I die

Will I no longer cry?

Will I escape the hurtful lies?

When I die will I fly?

Moments Of Contemplation

Cigarettes…

Soul searching as I stare at the sky

That holds clouds of questions

The answers whisper on the midnight breeze

Why is there sadness?

Whatever happened? To morning hugs and goodnight kisses?

All fleeting desires floating in the night of doubt

I'm a cowboy riding my stallion named rebellion

To the loving arms of inner peace

Music sunshine happy thoughts…

Mining the gold for my life's road

2008

Feelings locked in a cage

Rage my true feelings locked in a cage

The key held by my shadow hammer & coffin

Nails no drugs 'n alcohol but addicted

To that nervous twitch looking 4 a fight

Feeling like it's my right rite of passage

Those 'round me see me smile rarely

Anger's been my constant companion

Ally 'n teacher I love my mother but

My chains won't let me reach her

Arguments and verbal darts I instigate

And throw iz there another way

If there iz I don't know how to

Reach it peace I seek it another

Path but 2 many bridges burn to travel

It harsh words 'n bad decisions it will

Take the hand of god holding my heart 'n soul

2 heal it console it music 'n cigarettes

Medication but my anger they can't defeat

This Goliath David with bare knuckles

If I don't wise up I'm in trouble

Walking the edge of a 2 sided

Blade am I insane? Always looking 4

The pain in love this crutch I

Can no longer lean on

Oh how deceiven' my friend has been

You betray lead me astray there is

Only this I can say in my defense

I will try to go 4th hence to a place

Without these demons where I feel safe.

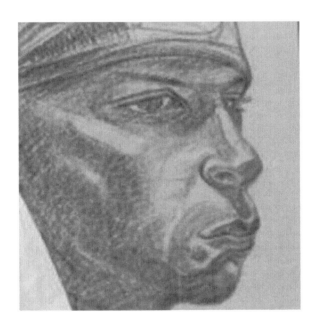

A Look in the Mirror

My life though better, still feel pressure

Clouds over my head these be the truest

Words I've said sunshine I ain't

Seen in a long time the path I'm on

Dark and uncertain feel like I'm in

A sad play but never seen behind

Drawn curtains my family stands

Beside me however I don't understand

Me C-R-Y-I-N-G always trying

To advance still stuck in a trance

Of anger's dance depressed oh how

I wish I was on greener pastures

And not feel like a bastard so

Many things I've said that hurt so

Many I tread over hot lava my own

Demons continue to suffer me

Can't let go of what I was is it

Because I refuse my pride won't let me

Lose but still I feel defeated

Have I conceded that it's to a

Dark place I'm headed so many

Thoughts never expressed like how I still

Feel loneliness past stress I've done

My wrongs I confess but that

Was then must I still pay for my

Sins? One year sober and clean

But so many things I haven't and still

Wish to see a Love Scene

I longed for but so confused

In my soul's core feel torn

By the two sides that reside

In my head and my heart

What part should I listen to?

I want to love you but still don't love

Myself want to trust you but still don't trust myself

My past struggles still feel like shackles

Situations seem so difficult to tackle

I wonder is this just an example

Of a path less travelled?

Where I came from and lives I've lived

Tear and rip at my being will I ever

Wear a wedding ring? Be a father?

If I do will I be like my

Stepfather? My mom's husband

When I was born nightmares in daydreams

Leave me forlorn it's not fair

My life should have been easier

Dealing with FAS never being with

My real father Doug Mann

I'm so sorry we never really talked

Maybe one day we will walk

Like Dad and kid like we should've did

I mean why should've James come

Between us never gave us a chance to love

Each other and to my brothers

I miss you Ronnie and Jimmy I love you

I'm so proud I'm an uncle

Ronnie you lost your kids to the same

Situation that we went through

Though I'm not there I'll pray for you

To my mom Christine a queen

So pristine no matter what

You taught me it's okay

To be me you gave me up and I

Can't even begin to imagine how

Tough that must have been

You want me to come home

You must be so alone your second child

In another province but I believe

In providence that one day

We will be reunited you did no wrongs

You brought me into existence gave me

The gift of life just knowing that was

Worth all the strife Thunder

Bay fifteen to nineteen a crazy scene

Away from the SCRCBC *

So sorry for the times I dissed you

Helen and Robert

Every time I fight all I want to do

Is stop it too many times apart

I remember that first night

In that house on Wharf I cried

And didn't sleep wary of

Snakes that would creep

I almost let D and A overtake me

I almost let my own fear and pain

Forsake me I still regret every time

I let my rage overtake me

You don't deserve the hurt of harsh

Words spoken my heart feels broken

As I think of all the times I

Chose to use or drink instead

Of letting you close I needed you

Then and still need you I have

So many issues so many tear soaked

Cheeks and wet tissues I've said

So much but it feels like not enough

I'm not tough enough to do it alone

The family quilt still waiting to be sewn

I want to be there when you need me

Like you do for me raised me

And rescued me too many times to count

I love you and from the tallest building

I will shout I can't see myself

Making it without you W.H.O

Wotton Halet Oswald I'm proud of our world.

February 2010

Sunshine Coast Roberts Creek British Columbia

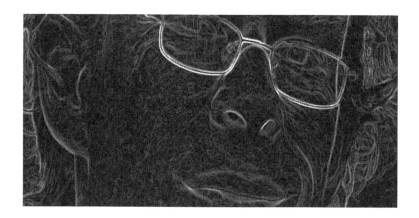

Warm Heart & Cold Coffee

(a country and western song)

VERSE ONE

The rain of that September morning was beating down like a
drum I don't know how, but I slept right through it she was
up when I walked in the kitchen yawning,

CHORUS

With a warm heart and cold coffee and a smile on her face, the
softness of her housecoat on my skin loving me with a kiss
and a good mornin' It was the best one I ever had with a
warm heart and cold coffee.

VERSE TWO

We both lay on the porch swing and stared at the sky not one
word spoken 'tween us two In that moment I felt more alive
than anytime in my life

CHORUS

With a warm heart and cold coffee and a smile on her face, the warmth of her housecoat on my skin loving me with a kiss and a good mornin' It was the best one I ever had with a warm heart and cold coffee.

BRIDGE

There could've been a hurricane and the whole world might've changed but lost in her arms I doubt I would've noticed a thing....

September 12th 2010

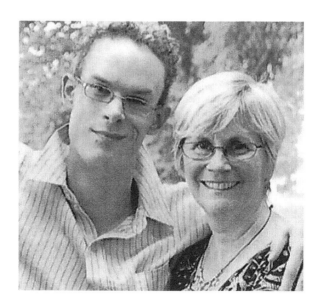

Dearest Soldier

It's your mom. Stay safe. Look both ways.

It's your dad. Remember, takes more than fighting to be a man.

It's your grandma and grandpa. Make it back safe for the extra treats, like ice cream and staying up late.

It's your aunt and uncle. Love, laugh and smile.

It's your son. Please come home. I can't play catch alone.

It's your daughter. A girl needs her mom and dad for life when it's good and when it's bad.

It's your wife. A vow was spoken. Please, through this unfair sickness, make it back in good health.

It's your husband. The pillows are getting harder to hold.

It's your sister. It's your brother. I miss you so, summer feels cold as winter.

It's your cousins, great and distant, 1st 2nd 3rd. Heed our words…the ribbons mean we support you our tears scream we miss you.

It's your nephew. It's your niece. If you're looking for peace, it's us kissing your cheek.

It's your grandson. It's your granddaughter. A kid needs their grandpapa and grandmamma.

It's your girlfriend. With my love, my heartache I send.

It's your boyfriend. When will this hell ever end?

It's your friends, buddies pals and chums. One for all and all for one! BFF!

It's the one writing you this letter,

Make it home. Please don't leave all these precious people sad and alone.

Rain Falling From The Morning Sky

Inspiration washing away the questions that I'm asking

As I hear it tap the ground around me

Once was I blind, walking backwards down the path set

before me

Now, my eyes wide, the rain falls freely

Cleansing my soul

My mind's eye holds that rain

In the form of tears, ridding me of doubt and fear

Yes the sunshine is sublime, but in a rainy scene

I find myself serene, my strength renewed

I cry, yes indeed I do my friend, for your pain

For my pain I do the same

Why must I dwell in this self-imposed cage anymore?

I walk now, feet on the ground

Won't you take my hand across the land

Over any obstacle whatever spectacle some might see

Beyond any judgments by others or ourselves

This has to be heaven cuz it don't rain happy tears in hell.

AIRPLANES PART 3

(Adapted from Airplanes by B.O.B. and Haley Williams of Paramore and Eminem)

VERSE ONE

Let's pretend that it's not the way it is or the way it was in my past being born without FASD had a normal childhood with my mom and my dad was not forced away and I could feel his love like I did not go from home to home from an infant to year 6 Let's pretend I was a happy kid so carefree never had to deal with any bullies High school I graduated was not made to feel hated I think of this when I see an airplane in the heavens...

VERSE TWO

Let's pretend I did not find writing exciting like I never had a way to say what was going on with me like I never saw tragedy or if I did I never picked up a pen or a pencil and scribed words that were genuine and real like my life was a movie and we removed the reel what would it have been like to have the name Mike and never once dreamed of rocking the Mic at 13 did not enter that talent show and allowed my love for hip hop to show no paper ever heard my name and I was sending wishes to chase airplanes

VERSE THREE

Let's pretend when I was addicted it was the end my sickness shakes cold sweats messy clothes unkempt crack cocaine and Jim Beam my only companions never grew out of that to become this champion and with every hit of the pipe or bottle I was sending out prayers full throttle

VERSE FOUR

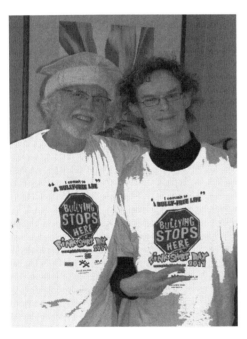

Let's pretend that it is the way it is that I'm a complex man who grew from a hard living kid I was rescued at a tender age by a loving woman and man who are the sole reason for my words on this page and yeah I went from heaven to hell more than once but there are so many I love and I trust I have so much ahead for me in my life I daydream all d-a-y and I don't have to scan the s-k-y for 747's or Cessna's.

HERE I LIE

Here I lie
In a bed full of questions
On a pillow of wonder
Covered by a quilt of "what if's?"

My mind
Rewinds times all time
Fast forwards infinitely
Much too fast
For simply me

The eggs have been counted
And put in the basket
The ducks are in a row
Ready for tonight's dinner
Of certainty?

The Saints
No, not football at all
Mary, Joseph, Michael
Wouldn't it be great if we

Could hear and see them all

Ask anything receive answers

Clear as a crystal globe

December 8, 2011

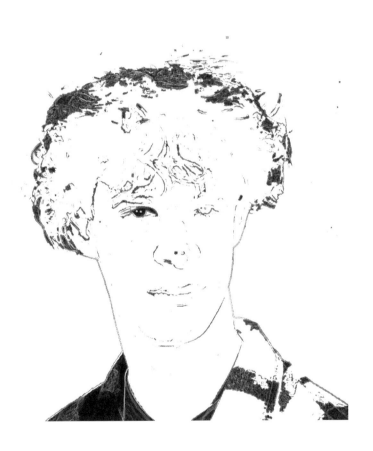

Runaway (But 2 where)

I could leave this place but to what end?

Would it justify the means of all my unspoken thoughts and
utter mistakes?

I could just pick up and go against the flow of the raging river
that drowns me. Where to however?

Is it my true nature? Every tie that suits me I sever

 4 just a little extra pleasure?

God knows I want 2 run away (but 2 where?)

A Joke with a Never Ending Punch Line

Is my life a parody?

The riddle in a fable as I walk down my coal brick road?

I scrape my hands to bone digging for diamonds

Only to have them turn to dust, as I hear a distant laugh.

Will this sick riddle ever be solved? Or is my life

A Joke with a Never Ending Punch Line?

Why?

 A question if I may.

Why do you and why do I not find the answers that will break
open the prison of perceptions that are held over us like so
many black clouds?

Why must so many seek a quick fix?

Like me, when I act on the judgments that blind me.

My own house of mirrors is a hall of illusions.

Why do I smash the glass and welcome the bad luck?

Slicing me like the knives in my back placed there by my own

hand?

Truth Soul Armour

Feelings inside.

Soul confused.

Am I up when I'm so down?

My mind won't let me 4get my missteps.

A cruel twist of fate that battles me at the start of every

mourning of the peace of mind heart and soul.

Each day I pick up the shattered pieces of my

Truth ~ Soul ~ Armor

January 5, 2012

a sonnet

Alone I danced one day upon the shore

My feet were cold to raging wind

I shivered almost to my core

Orange sky held painted tinge

my cold toes caressed the waves

yet the day felt like the rest

each step I turn another page

in my head I sing my utmost best

music moving through my hands

fingers tracing notes in silence

my body seems to understand

all beauty without violence

dancing night and day away

I would have it no other way

January 16, 2012

Poems Time Spent

On The Phone…

Six Zero Four

A beginning

To a conversation

One with the woman I love

Eight Eight Five

Closer ever so closer

To hearing her voice again

The voice of my blond haired rose

The next four numbers

A closely guarded secret

A code to my heart

A numerical sequence

That is as natural as breathing

"Hello?" comes her voice

I take a breath feeling blessed once more

"Hey!"

I reply.

Listening to music…

Plug in my Marc Ecko headphones

Slide the musical vessels on my ears

Turn on my iPod

Tune out the world

What shall it be?

Rather who shall it be?

Country? Rap? Metal?

Or maybe R&B?

Whatever genre I choose

Such joy at my fingertips

Such an assortment

Of talent

…a hard decision

2Pac, Trey Songz, Stitchez or Mars?

Or maybe none of the above

Perhaps sweet songs of love

By Evanescence or Kenny Chesney

Songs I can croon too

Words that make me cry

Rhymes I have memorized

Like a computer plugged into a computer

I am with my music

An encyclopedia of knowledge

Discographies and song titles

Years of release and features

I will love music now

And forever in the future.

Working On The Computer...

Open my Asus laptop

Pressing the power ON

I am close

To my connection

My center

Of circuits

Children of the motherboard

I hear the song greeting me with my desktop imagery

What is it I choose today for such a layout?

A rapper? A car? Oh, I know, SPORTS!

I click on Internet Explorer

I am open to the net now

Open to the net, what a concept for a line of poetry

If I am involved with a net am I not caught?

That would explain countless hours spent

Back to my inter dimensional experience

I am my homepage

A page of my choosing

To begin my journey

W W W dot

Google dot com

I click on images

I type

My fingers dancing on the keys to some unheard beat

Basketball

a picture of the Celtics of Boston jersey

AHA! I shout, perfect choice!

Left click with the right hand, for I have only one option left

Set as background to my next time of being caught

In the net.

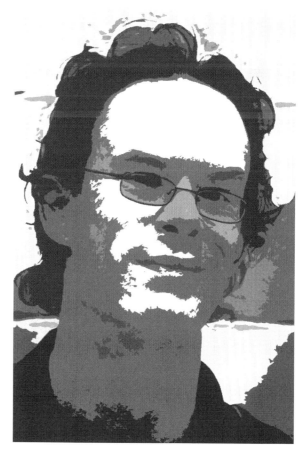

Without Music

Without music

I am deaf

Without words I am blind

Without control

I am unleashed inside

A raging implosion

Set to go off on a hair trigger

Thinner than the air itself

Just try to disarm me

But beware of the dog

And its teeth to the hand

Working that sensitive nerve circuit

Bitten never to be sewn

My utter rage

Now quite known

Throw me a bone

I will stand up and bark proudly

As I string you up

And you choke and sputter

Gasp and perish

And hang you on display

To be witnessed by your parish

Now I am
AM FM
Once agnostic
Now seeking religion
Trigger self-disarmed
Dog napping
Barking softly as in dream
I am in control
I have hold of your hand
In mine as they embrace
Erasing all pain
Leaving no trace

February 6, 2012

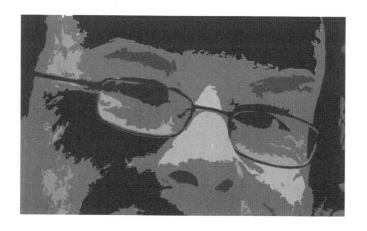

SYMBOLISM POEMS

1. Mirror

I look into the mirror

I see myself, but not quite myself

My body is surrounded by a darkness I cannot see

For the darkness is the past inside of me

2. Sky

The sky

So wild and free

Just like my soul

My mind

My body

3. World

The world

So full of fear and rage

I feel like I am locked in a cage

I wish I knew what to do

To make it better for me and you

February 9, 2012

Youth

ONE ASKED THE OTHER
"How can I?"
"What could I do?"
I pondered with a shrug.

"Give a helping hand
It's better than a drug
Give a hug!"

"Dig in your wallet
For that $20 bill
Instead of allowing your pockets to fill"

Donate
Appreciate
Participate
 Turn away?
That's just fear

Stand by our side
We need you here.

Free Form from Titles

A Day in the Life

AM
Eyes open
Awaiting taste of coffee
Mouth savouring
Sounds of music from IPod
Body dressed
In plans for the day
Anoint myself with oils of
"I AM OK"

NOON
Day half gone
Glass half full
Top it up with
Smiles and laughs
Errands run and events partaken
Drape myself in radiant sunshine
On days of dark clouds
And rain days I dance

PM
Evening now
Day gone
Glass still sits full
I sit with my family
Three Knights of the Round Table
Our noble beast purrs, meows, and dances
Between our legs
We sit, full of halves and beginnings
Ready for the entrée of wholes

Now I sit in bed
Music reflecting my life at today's point
Now my eyes close
Till tomorrow rolls around.

ONE WORD AT A TIME

Write there is no wrong
Pen I am free
I sit on my cil and watch the day go by
Daydreams never give way
To nightmares
Too much to look forward to
I am but a vessel
In this ocean of literary possibility
Eye See You Sea-ing me
Is it an error or another point of view?
Only we can find the solution
One Word At a Time.

TIME TO LISTEN

As the clock ticks
My ears perk up
Waiting to discover the jewels
In your words
Their drums beating a song of joy
At the angelic music that is your voice
On the cell or home phone
Or in 3D in front of me
Never shall I turn a blind eye
For I shall then forever have a deaf ear
And I would suffer
Never hearing you again
And lose my time to listen.

WALK IN MY SHOES

Micheal Oswald Mann
A man yet a man
Journey with me
Walk a path
Of love and pain
Sorrow and joy
Tears and laughter
Sometimes the previous two
Intermingle in times of complete joy
Like now thinking of all I have
Tears of joy
Filling me
Pouring out
Fly with me now
Beyond the dawn
As I drift away
Like evanescence
Pain when it comes
Hurts like a hundred lashes
Stinging me ever a constant reminder
To stay on the path of the righteous Mann
The boy I spoke of earlier
The part of me carrying humour
And the tears of joy and the fall
Of sorrow so much unresolved
Puzzle yet to be solved
Burning like a solvent
I crawl in my convent
To be angry
Is too convenient
Marred by thee
Thee Thy Me
Mine own hand
Reaches for thine,
Reaches for yours.

Walk in my shoes I ask of you never
For only I can finish this journey.

March 5, 2012

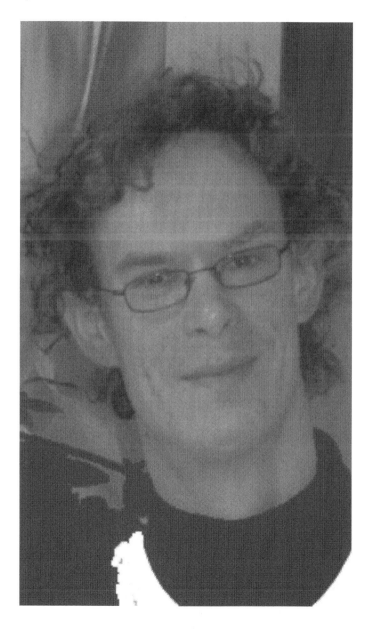

A POEM FOR KEVIN

A smile on your face

There never was a day

When you didn't laugh

You brought my spirits high

But now I only cry

I am so sad

Though I can be glad

That I knew you

I feel your spirit here

You are not really gone

I see your twinkling eyes

In the sunshine

And the Moonlight

I see you

And I smile

Kevin, brother, buddy, pal, you were a friend to me

You may be on the other side

But the tide still ebbs

Time still flows

And I feel woe

But I will take the other road

I will try to laugh like you

To smile like you

And be a friend like you

I am a better human being

Because I knew you...

Kevin, This prayer I send for you....

Lord, when you see an angel at your gates, with a twinkle in his eye and a smile on his face, let him in to your grace.

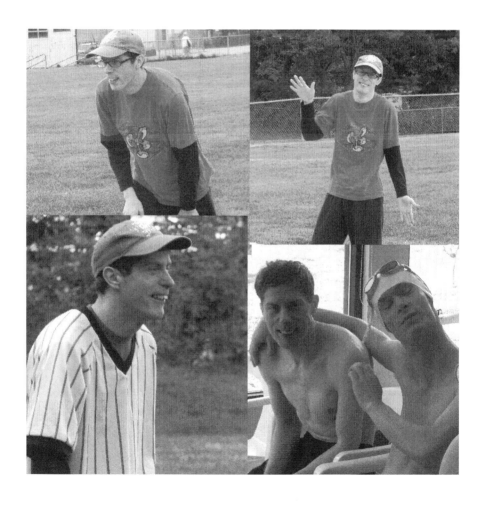

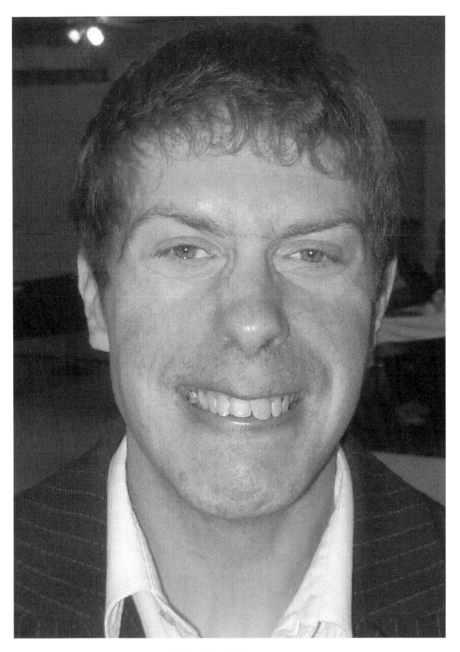

Kevin Norman

February 15, 1978 – October 22, 2010

Dearest Mr. Grumpy,

I want you to know that I realize the hurt and pain you have felt for so long.

I am here to console you. No longer will you be alone. In the past I let you go off with no guidance.

I know now that with my newfound faith in you that together we can become Micheal and Mr. Happy.

I, Micheal Douglas Mann want you to understand that the past is the past and it's not happening now nor will it ever.

In times of need I can take your hand in mine and let you know with care and love that it's all gonna be ok.

Today marks a new dawn in our friendship, friends looking out for friends with love and care. Any concerns we have the power to overcome, and any obstacle can be hurtled over with a purpose and positive energy.

Mr. Happy is now your name. The mocking moniker of your past is no more.

I Love You Mr. Happy.

Sincerely,

Micheal Douglas Mann.

Mon, Apr 23 2012

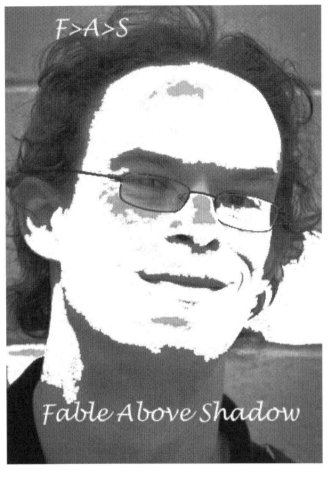

F>A>S

Fable Above Shadow

03/15/1982

on this time of earth's existence/ born a prince/ the man in the iron mask/ put to task/ survived the wrath/ of all put before me/ lived each sunrise/ as a warrior with a general's pride/ like an army residing within me/ f.a.s./ fable above shadow/ once thought a mere story/ now my presence is undeniable/ my body draped in the finest apparel/ my mind that of Lucifer's child/ at first glance/ I may appear a normal being/ I tell you now/ that's complete misunderstanding/

my future conquests already scribed on a sacred scroll/ in the age of King Arthur at his round table/ I let my daily life guide me and be my teacher/ the words I trust spoken by the heat of the sun/ mother/ father/ sisters/ brothers/ friends and precious loved ones/ with every coming of the moon/ I grow stronger/ I knew in infancy/ that the galaxy would be my home no longer/ I am meant for a greater destiny/ with truth of mind/ to drive me/ my song will be sung by the afterfathers/ with great sincerity/ tales of conquering/ all that is thought implied/ when spoken my name/ when false prophets speak with misfortune and disdain/ I've felt the sharpest of flames/ marched through the chilling of the coldest rains/ now you may read this passage/ and think oh how pompous/ but I had to shed light of truth on deceitful darkness/ fought with the bravest of women and men/ only the first billion years can be put to paper/ with this noble pen/ I shall exist long after what you think of as universe ceases/ I leave this authentication/ for you to read this.

RAPS

"... without rap in my life..."

Note to Readers: If you aren't used to reading rap, it helps a lot to read it out loud.

When You See Me

When you see me/ how do you perceive?/ fool/ fake/ some
kind of wanna be?/ do you see/ me as an actor/ like I belong
on TV?/ I want to let you know/ I live for hip-hop's flow and
ebb/ the culture full integrated/ in me/ engrained in my
mannerisms/ and my speech/ without rap in my life/ I
wouldn't have half of what I write/ so before you judge/ call
me a wigger and such/ recognize/ the truth I describe/ this
music/ and sub genres/my life blood/ I am more than just
some punk/ this rap game's got me locked for years and
months/ I identify/with verses/ lyrics and hooks/ even
though myself am no crook/ my own style/ leaves
disbelievers shook/ maybe/ I won't end up doing/ h-i-p/ r-a-
p/ h-o-p/ but forever shall it be/ a full and engrained source
of me/ got love for all true mc's/ backpackers/ to thugs rollin
trees/ real is my/ realit/ tie/ ever hunger/ rye

2012

yo/ yo/ check it out one time/ for ya freaked out mind/ I spit a rhyme/ so complex/ intricate/ like a spider's web/ but nowhere as delicate/ solid/ like titanium/ off the top of my cranium/ medulla/ oblongata/ my brain/ mind going insane/ with this/ gift/ to spit/ piff/ wickedly/ sincerely/ yo it mikey/ m to the I to k to e to the/ y do I spell my name?/ so won't forget it/ expanding my fame/ got game/ mad lyrics circling/ my fingers/ touching the keyboard/ so hot/ keys are sizzling/ what is up?/ the sky/ and this b-boy guy/ twenty/ nine/ with an adamantium spine/ so kind I can be/ a gentleman/ sweet as pastry/ tick me off/ I go off/ the rail/ don't be around/ me/ at that time section/ or get an injection of me seeing red/ me wanting bloodshed/ or destruction of day/ and proper/ tay/ I am learning how to act/ more appropriately/ this rap I write/ I am finding delight/ in the sole factor/ in this art/ I am a master/ of ceremony/ some call it MC/ microphone/ controller/ style so hot/ call it solar. Why are/ things the way/ they are/ why me/ I ask/desperately/ I scream in fact/ I try not to over/ react/ love mixed/ with feeling like ish/ holding back/ words that/ though honest/ could damage/ my relationship/ confused which path/ to choose/ I try my best/ best/is all I can do/ my girl/ I/love/ you/ I/ miss/ you/ need to be/ near you/ I hope I'm not too clingy/ fear losing my soul to the truth/ are we ever going to be/ mr and mrs?/this is what/I am/hopin'

A Rap for my Mom

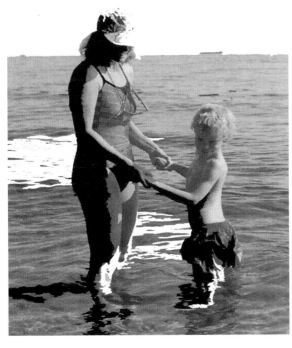

Been with my momma for two decades/ and change/ now I have to explain/ can't refrain/ from representing/ all the times she/ hugged/ and loved/ me/ wiped tears from my eyes/ made me smile/ not cry/ rescued me from bad/ situations/ dark locations/ supported every dream/ with constructive/ criticism/ there are not enough/ isms/ to express my/ dedication/ my mami/ seen all sides of me/ the one I'm showing/ is the one about loving/ and knowing/ she gives it back/ with no fronting/ I gotta take a sec/ to say my regrets/ for any disrespect/ merci beau coup/ for keeping me in check/ if I could/ I would/ give you everything you dream/

but I know your love/ for me/ can't amount to any cream/ my momma/ moms/ and mom/ this here flow/ is direct/ from your son/ with love/ you sweet as a rose/ beautiful as a dove.

Rap for My Dad

My dad/ the only one I every knew/ who stuck by my side/ stayed honest and true/ I love him/ for his support/ he sees my goals and says go for it!/ I don't know what I'd do without/ a man to help me out/ when I need that father to son chat/ you know/ 'bout this/ 'bout that/ guy stuff/ sometimes things are tough/ but we always seem to overcome/ working in the yard/ me and him/ reading story/ so many times spent/ pure and glory/ filled/ my pops keeps it real/ 100 per cent/ and like I've said/ we've had our bumps in our road/ I get mad/ we explode/ but never mind that/ cuz this ain't about that/ it's 'bout the sacred pact/ made 'tween man and son/ I believe our journey's just begun/ can't wait/ I know he'll be great/ as/ a/ grand/ pa to my little ones/ one day/ what more can I say?/ he's there rock solid all the time/ I love R Dub so much/ I wrote this rhyme.

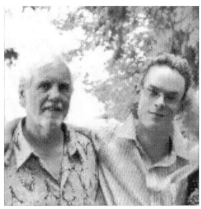

Rap for a Woman

Hey queen/ to talk truth/ you're a goddess/ your beauty goes beyond/ your body or the way you dress/ my desire goes/ far beyond sex/ I was just wondering/ if you/ would just give me a few/ to chat with you/ get to know you/ what your needs be/ and what are your wants?/ it's been so long since I felt like this/ I may be thuggish/ but sensitive/ I know your feelings must be tentative/ so don't let me rush/ I wanna see your soul with my mind/ not my finger's touch/ this moment is a stroke of luck/ just sitting having this convo/ you got my heart locked like five oh/ you are just so exceptional/ funny, gorgeous/ an acclaimed intellectual/ so much I know/ but you hold the truth/ I have sought for/ all my years/ been with a few girls/ but you are a woman/ right here/ I thank you for sharing this time/ if we meet again/ it might be a sign/ til then keep doing what you're doing/ gracias for being/ sweet/ caring and gracious.

INTROSPECTIVES TO A PAST LIFE

I sit here/on my bed/feeling dread/ of tomorrow/ knowing that no toke or drink/ will choke/ or drown sorrow/ My mom and dad ask/ what's wrong?/ so let me explain/ best I can in this song/ I'm twenty five/ feel I waste life/ alone/ no numbers in my cell phone/ I smile but tears come/ I see all I got/ which I admit is a lot/ here's where the plan gets unfortunate/ love/ I live without it/ pain's my best friend/ will he be here/ till the end/ my shadow is the only one who laughs at my jokes/ is my life a joke?

You wish to ridicule me/ cuz I'm a man with a disability/ with dreams of being an MC/ I speak in rhyme/ though no one hears me/ I cry tears/ yet no one sees them/ I think about sleeping pills/ taking all of them/ with a six pack of Heineken/ or maybe cutting my wrists/ Anything better/ than to wake up like this/ you say you know me/ do you/really?

I speak with sincerity/ in a desperate/ futile search/ for serenity/ all caught up in serendipity/ with no clear view/ or window to look through/ I dare not laugh/ like I am the youngest and only survivor in a car crash/ there are those around me/ who love/ and care for me/ when they leave/ or I do/ I feel lousy/ split in two/ one side high/ trying not to cry/ the other/ missing my father/ and mother/ breaking down in the street/ at all the weary miles/ on these tired feet.

The word on the street/ is I'm the laughingstock/ keep up the talk/ I shall rise above/ or at least I will try/ don't be surprised/ if I am young/ when I meet/my demise/ I spend wasted hours wasted/ drunk/ high/ buzzed or half cut/ my willingness to stand has been struck down/ soul sucked out/ how long/ till I recite these words/ to God/ when I do/ will he cry or applaud?
2005

Dear World,

I'll be gone soon/ from a wound/ self inflicted/ led a life/
stressful/ conflicted/ twenty five/ can't see a future/ in my/
mind's eye/ loved ones/ do not cry/ and this is why/ no
more pain I'll feel/ when my casket is sealed/ so many
mistakes/ broken promises made/ shook hands with the
devil/ made a deal/ accepted all errors corrected/ so please/
just bury me/ I feel all the pain/ from you all/ I had to make/
this fate/ ful choice/ to break/ my fall/ otherwise/ I would
stay eternally/ hypnotized/ by false hope/ in a world that
only/ knows/ how to cry/and deny hope/ for its/
inhabitants/ so plant me in the earth/ after driving the
hearse/ to the cemetery/ I do not find this situation/ scary/
with the razor to my wrists/ I no longer feel I need to/
persist/ to wish/ any luck/ it's all fucked up/ brain knows
nothing/ but how to screw up/so away I go/ to heaven or
hell/ I do not quite know/ when you close your eyes/ you
will see me/ assuring thee/ of my sincerity/ that no longer
will you have to simply tolerate/ or put up with me/ I'm
gone/ no pain/ no problems/ .44 to my dome/ soon the other
side/ will be home.

2005

BALANCE

I want balance in my life/ my mentality/ is instability/
wanna be/ the mc/ who has recognition/ purpose in his
position/ pisces in opposite directions/ dreams in differential
sections/ cash to live on/ legacy to live on/ skills to rely on/
willing to work on/ my technique/ technician/ working/ on
brain circuitry/ left for creative purposes/ right/ for write/
ing/ down these prophetic verses/ don't want to be/ the next
Slim Shady/ big cars/ tons of ladies/ screw that cuzzin/ cuz/
I don't need to spit about crack or gats busting/ cuz that ain't
me/ soul is/ p-u-r/ e/ situations/ with pads/ and pens/ lead
me/ to victory/ I look to be not stressful/ strictly peaceful/
writing like a painter on an easel B.I.G/ P.A.C/ some of the
mc's/ that influence me/ my melody sweet like a note/ by
MJB/ Rap and hip hop till I be/ deceased/ from night/ to/
day/ cuz one thing you gonna say/ yo remember son?/ skills
he got on...

Why I listen to Horrorcore

(Please understand that I in no way whatsoever condone any of the actions lyrically portrayed in horrorcore rap.)

I choose to listen to horrorcore for many reasons. For example, for a short period of time as a young child, I watched horror movies constantly. I quickly became a fan of this movie genre as it was the main type of movie playing at my home. I enjoy listening to rap music. It was a natural progression to horrorcore once I discovered it, because I was (and still am) a fan of horror movies as an adult.

All artists in this genre are 100% independent and are not under major label pressure. This allows for the taboo subject matter, as well as original and innovative styles and ideas. I agree with this because I revel in the fact that no one can tell these artists what they can or cannot say, as they do not suck up to A&R's for money or radio play, depending on word of mouth and a loyal fan base. This makes the music rare and hard to find. I like this because I know of only a handful of people who know of the same artists I listen to.

As hip hop/rap is worldwide, so is horrorcore. I listen to artists from Russia, Sweden, Australia etc. This shows me that horrorcore is worldwide and internationally known. You can say the same for all music I know, but it thrills me nonetheless.

For me, when I look for horrorcore to listen to, I have my faves. Sicktanick, Razakel, Stichez(r.i.p) Stitchmouth, Necro, Kidcrusher, Dyad Souls, Q-Strange, Boondox...I really could go on and on...

I enjoy female horrorcore artists a lot because they take what it means to be a woman and in a sense, turn it on its head. Razakel for example, speaks about female serial killers on her album Femicide, a term used to describe murder of women, but she takes the word and flips it.

I am a church going, bible reading, praying Christian so one might ask, "Why do you listen to this?" I will tell you why. I choose to listen to horrorcore because I enjoy the dark subject matter, it's like totally opposite to how I practice my day to day life, so I consider it a way to explore my dark side.

There is a story told about two wolves. One is a white wolf, the other black. One represents happiness and love, the other anger and hate. They are constantly in battle. The question is which one wins? The one you feed is the answer.

I choose to feed both wolves, and to dabble in my dark side because I am fascinated by this original sub genre, for reasons that I will get into now.

We all have a dark side. Whether we choose to acknowledge it is up to any individual. For me, hearing Sicktanick rap about the occult thrills me, as I am also a Christian. It's almost like I shouldn't listen, yet I do anyway.

Call me a hypocrite if that makes you feel better, you could say I am not a true Christian if you wanted to, but in reply to that I would say you are judging me and you have no right. I don't preach occultism to my fellow church members, I don't murder people because a rap artist talks about it, I know the difference between music and reality thank you very much.

So there is your answer to the question...why do I listen to horrorcore? Cuz I like it. It thrills me. It's dark and I enjoy my dark side as well as my light side. Can't have one without the other!

Pce out!
February 2, 2012

In Conclusion

Life

Each day at sunrise/ we arise/ shrugging off what we can of strife/ heal pains of agony and heartbreak that cuts like knives/ our lives/ so complex/ questions not enough/ equals plus troubles are multiplied by all we add and subtract love/ hate laugh cry/ always why/ the eternal question/ but shall I mention tidbits of all we seek/ gathered by appreciation of the meek/ and lessons of the mighty?/ AM to PM first star I wish on is the same/ I first glance upon the moon out in day/ time ever remind/ ing us of continuum of time/ and tides/ till I in peace rest/ must endure pleasures and pain/ and all the rest/ my chest/ contains my heart/ my head my mind/ my body my soul/ those who stand by me/ warm me/ when I'm cold/ starve my fears/ feed me light/ letting me see/ in the absence of supposedly/ none/ my heart can be won/ but I am not one/ to be thought of as none/ however changing of peoples things places and thoughts/ silent behind faces/ I can't change or affect in this existence/ circumstances/ many devil led dances/ forgotten joys/ sad romances/ only a fragment/ of my entanglement/ false pride and unneeded entitlement/ the poorest man with the wisest mind/ is the richest with a golden mind/ a diamond mine/ of jewels more rare/ than human can wear/ the tear/ of me from myself I cry about/ when tears fall/ eye to southbound/ enrich the ground/ I stand upon/ planting seeds/ giving sun and life to a brighter light/ now when most needed/ all I've ignored/ now know should have heeded/ but regrets be not needed/ for each second I live/ laugh/ love/ remember more than I'll ever forget/ lines rehearsed/ props in place/ set the stage for the play/ of my today...

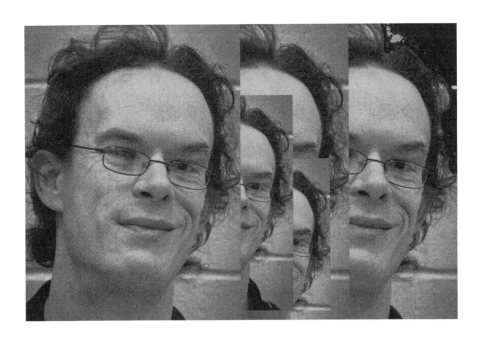

WITH APPRECIATION

To all those who gave advice/ guided me through life/ held my hand through the strife/ my love for you/ is totally/ and/utterly/ complete/ the talks I had with my mom/ her driving/ me/ in the/ passenger seat/ and hey dad/ you're rad/ always smiling/ even when/ I'm bad/ never changed/ your feelings/ kept it real/ never misleading/ I want you both there/ when Anthony hands me/ that wedding ring/ to you all/ this song I sing/ without you/ I don't know/where I'd be/ maybe/ 6 feet deep/ or the penitentiary/ thanks to all you all/ I know you're going to be there/ when I fall/ catching me/ helping me/ to understand/ the pleasures and pain/ of today's society/ I admit sometimes/ I stir up sh*t/ so I apologize/ from the bottom/ of my heart and soul/ you all/ all/ways/ kept my brain/ heart/ and belly full/ this is a heartfelt tribute/ you love me/ I love you/ from hand me downs/ to 100$ suits/ helping me /to appreciate/ the fruits/ of my labour/ if you need me/ I'll be/ there/ to rescue/ and save ya/ because I know you'd do so for me/ to others/ com ci/ com ca/ there's always karma/ this rhyme is not about ya/ it's those who were there/ whether/ I was/ north or south/ thanks for letting me sleep on the couch/ teaching me to stand proud/ not slouch/ have pride in who I am/

a young man/ appreciated and loved/ without you/ I'd be lost/ so thanks again/ for the lessons taught.

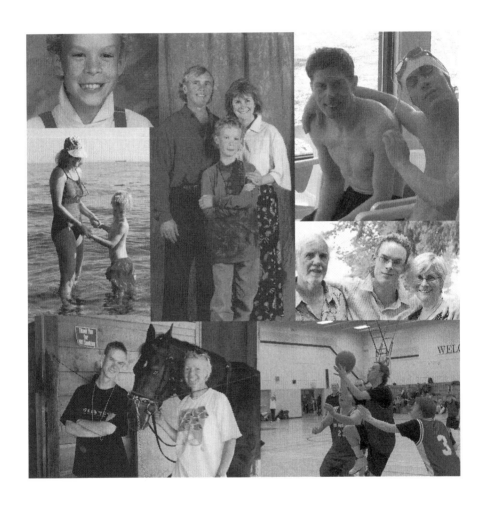

Dearest Readers,

I cannot tell you how overjoyed I am that you have read this book. At first I only wrote as a passion that came and went many times over. Now I am happy to be able to bring you ME; to bring Micheal D. Mann to life through my words.

I have covered a lot of ground in this book from FASD to my likes and hobbies, to my choices of music and entertainments, to my day-to-day life. I am so excited that you all went on this fabulous trip with me.

I can assure you this was certainly a daunting task, spanning many months, and to say it was an easy feat would be a fabrication. But it is most certainly a task I would take on again and again, as I am a writer, that's what we do.

I would also like to thank three incredible authors for guiding me on my journey as a writer: Jane Covernton, David Roche, and Heather Conn. David, from the beginning always encouraged me to further my talents. Heather worked endlessly on another book I hope to see in print one day, and certainly without Jane this book would not have been possible. My hat goes off to all of you. Thank you ever so much.

In closing this letter, I urge you to find that being inside each one of you that yearns to be heard and sit down with pencil or pen, paper or keyboard, and allow yourselves the freedom that writing brings. Or, for those who have other interests such as art, music, decorating, or crafting, push ahead with your gifts and allow yourself to shine. It will be most rewarding!!

Best regards,
Micheal D.Mann

Made in the USA
Charleston, SC
27 November 2012